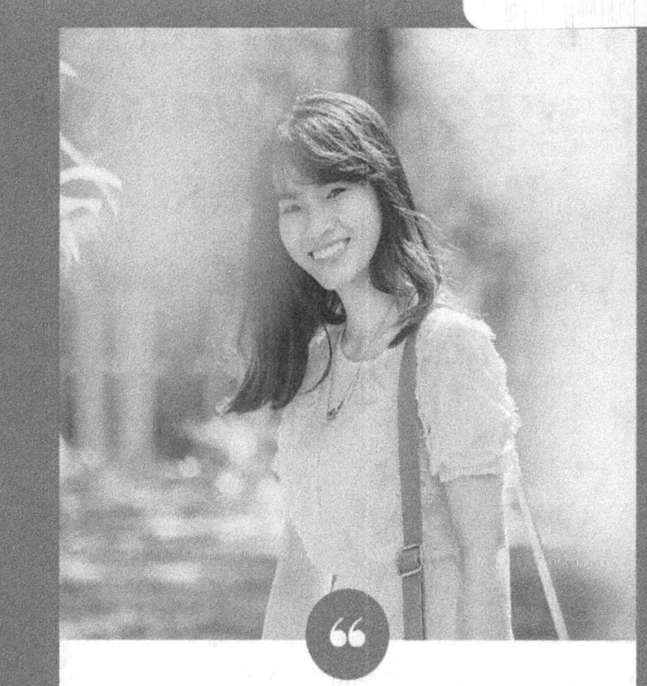

12 THINGS A SELF RESPECTING WOMAN WILL NEVER COMPROMISE ON

BEST SELLING FOR EVERY MAN & WOMAN

12 THINGS A SELF RESPECTING WOMAN WILL NEVER COMPROMISE ON

When a lady loves and respects herself she doesn't compromise with herself and with the merchandise she uses even in her relationship. Inexpensive objects are no longer solely exact for shallowness however for fitness too. It's better to spend more money than to lower your standards and health.

For example, a cheap make-up product can create some problems, a cheap mattress can spoil your posture, and lower-priced meals can make you unhealthy which can lead to extra expenses. So it is better to spend a little cash in the beginning than to spend it on making it good.

Meanwhile, among all the twelve things a respecting woman cannot compromise, the last in number is very important. So read to the end.

1. DRINKING WATER

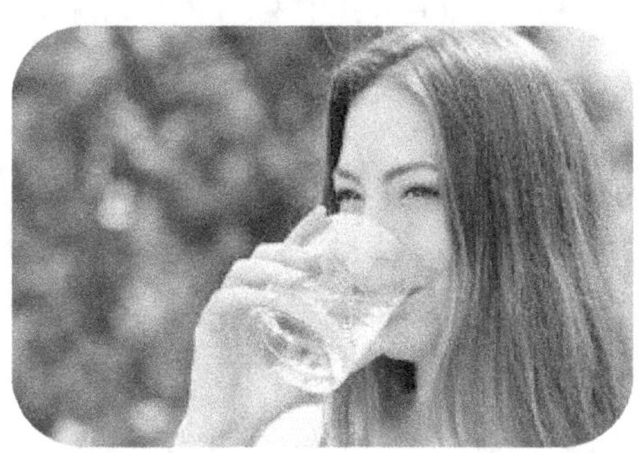

Clean water is necessary and must. Drinking faucet water that hasn't been boiled is risky and harmful. So keep away from consuming unhealthy and filthy water from somewhere and however a suitable bottle of mineral water.

Health Advantages Of Water To Woman

i.   It Helps Keep Skin Bright

Adequate water consumption will assist preserve your pores and skin hydrated and may additionally promote collagen production. However, water consumption alone isn't enough to minimize the consequences of aging. This technique is additionally linked to your genes and ordinary solar protection.

### ii.	It Helps Improve Mood

Not getting sufficient water can additionally affect your mood. Dehydration can also result in fatigue and confusion as nicely as anxiety.

### iii.	It Prevents Overall Dehydration

Dehydration is the result of your physique now not having ample water. And due to the fact water is quintessential to so many bodily functions, dehydration can be very dangerous.

Severe dehydration can result in a wide variety of extreme complications, including:

- swelling in your brain

- kidney failure

- seizures

Make positive you drink sufficient water to make up for what's misplaced thru sweat, urination, and bowel moves to keep away from dehydration.

iv.   It Aids In Cognitive Function

Proper hydration is key to staying in tip-top cognitive shape. Research Trusted Source suggests that now not consuming sufficient water can negatively affect your focus, alertness, and temporary memory.

v.   It Helps Boost Energy

Drinking water may additionally set off your metabolism. Improvement in metabolism has been related to a fine effect on strength level.

One finds out about discovered that ingesting five hundred milliliters of water boosted the metabolic price with the aid of 30 percent in each man and woman. These outcomes seemed to ultimate over an hour.

vi.   It Helps Fight Off Illness

Drinking sufficient water can assist stop certain medical conditions.

These include:

- constipation

- kidney stones

- exercise-induced asthma

- urinary tract infection

- hypertension

Water additionally helps you soak up essential vitamins, minerals, and vitamins from your food, which will expand your possibilities of staying healthy.

vii.   It Helps You Lose Weight

Studies have linked body fats and weight loss with ingesting water in each obese girl's trusted Source and women. Drinking extra water whilst weight-reduction plan and exercising can also just assist you to lose greater pounds.

viii.   It Improves Blood Oxygen Circulation

Water incorporates beneficial vitamins and oxygen to your whole body. Reaching your each day water consumption will enhance your circulation and have an advantageous influence on your basic health.

2.   GOOD QUALITY DESSERTS

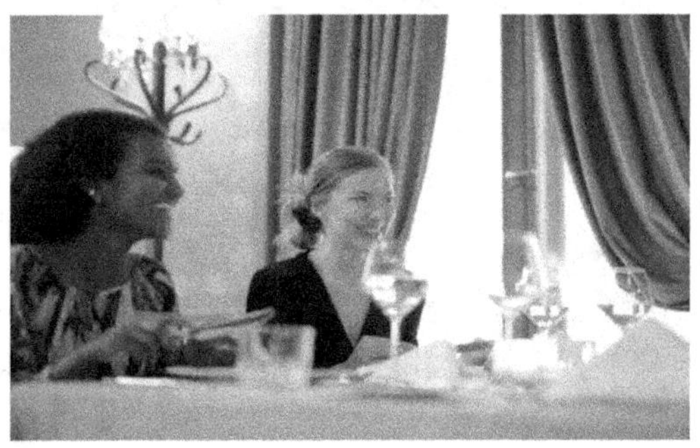

Desserts, chocolates, and women go together. Women love candies and sweets, they like to deal with themselves with the equal however save and neighborhood shop-bought matters are neither healthful nor hygienic.

Cutting sweets from your existence is no longer easy, so keep away from ingesting unhygienic and affordable pastries and sweets alternatively buy from some reputed save that affords healthful and fantastic cake and sweets.

Dessert is no longer solely delicious, however, it can help enhance your ordinary fitness and weight. Researchers from Tel Aviv University file that consuming dessert with breakfast, such as cookies or a slice of cake, can use resources with weight loss and assist preserve a wholesome lifestyle.

Benefits Of Eating Healthy

- Weight loss.

- Reduced cancer risk.

- Diabetes management.

- Heart fitness and stroke prevention.

- The health of the subsequent generation.

- Strong bones and teeth.

- Better mood.

- Improved memory

3.   THERMAL UNDERWEAR

Thermal underclothes is a kind of garb worn underneath your pinnacle layers to maintain your body warm, especially in the course of harsh iciness temperatures. Made from an area of expertise material to defend in opposition to the cold, women's thermal undies traps body warmth to provide warmth.

Thermal undies are the best. They don't appear vulgar and low-priced however seem to be classic. It will no longer solely make you seem cool however they hold us heat in winters. Thermal undies are the lengthy-time period funding in splendor and health. The mannequin relies upon upon the needs.

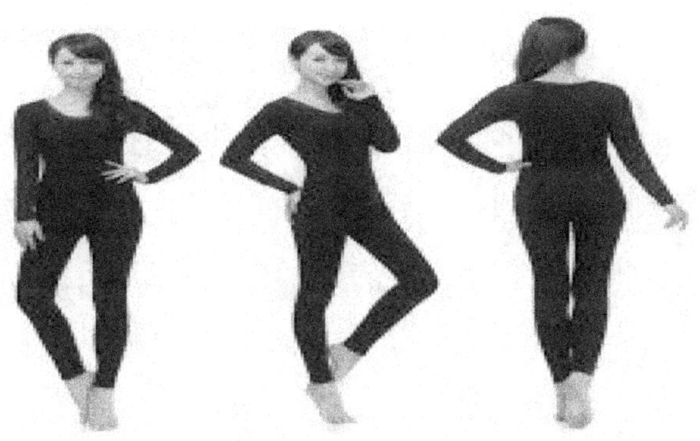

If you have a much less energetic life-style then you need to pick heat-saving underclothes made of wool and fleece. Moisture absorbing fashions are fantastic for humans who do a lot of bodily activities. And combined selections are exceptional for metropolis life.

You have to pick out the ideal dimension for you for greater benefits.

4.   HAIR DYING

Hair dying is in vogue these days. So take care whilst dying your hair. Besides the usage of a less expensive nice dye that is hazardous to the scalp and pores and skin use a precise first-rate dye for higher and wholesome results.

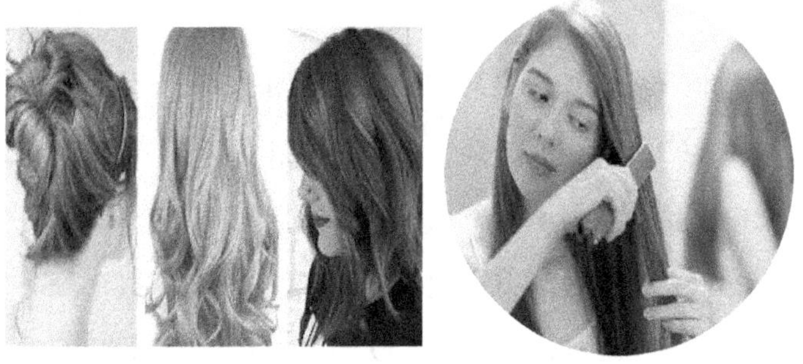

Hairs are an essential section of your beauty. So keep away from going to an amateur or anyone who isn't tons skilled due to the fact they can wreck your hairs too or you would possibly be apologetic about later after seeing the outcomes as a substitute go to an expert, ask for all the important points and then go for the loss of life for higher and satisfactory results.

For the female who selects to dye their hair, it is a way to exhibit off their style, their self-belief, and their personality. With a range of new hair shade tendencies surfacing, like opal, galaxy, pastel, and many more, extra females are selecting to exhibit off their real colors.

5.   HAND CARE

Hands are refined and the hands of a lady must be refined and soft. Well-groomed and tender arms exhibit how lots a lady takes care of herself. Your arms exhibit how a lot you care about yourself.

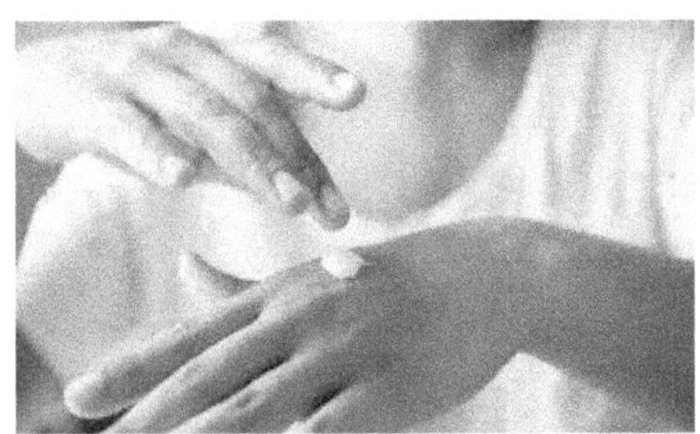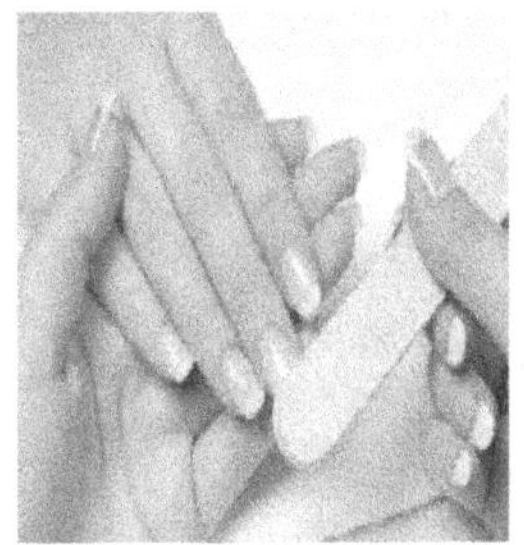

Taking care of palms is a must. You simply can't keep away from your palms and you should no longer think of saving your money. Grooming your fingers doesn't solely consist of the usage of a desirable and luxurious cream however taking applicable care and precautions like the use of gloves for cleansing and safety from the cold. Also, keep away from too much cold water and to a whole lot of hot water as washing your fingers with them can lead to cracks in your hands.

Why Is It Essential To Take Care Of Your Hands?

And absolutely everyone is constantly telling you the significance of washing your hands. In the direction of a day, your fingers are uncovered to all kinds of germs, dirt, harsh substances, daylight, and more. To make things worse, the common washing it is designed to maintain your fingers sanitary additionally can maintain them dry, cracked, and wrinkled.

Hand care and ideal hygiene is the single most essential way to forestall your self from getting ill and from spreading germs to others. 38% wash their fingers more than 10 times a day. ... It is essential to reflect on the consideration that moist hands are the wrongdoer for germs to spread.

6.   GOOD AND COMFORTABLE MATTRESS

A good and comfy mattress is a must for a fantastic posture of our body. A poorly chosen mattress can cause chronic pain and fatigue. It can additionally lead to negative posture. Manufacturers and doctors recommend altering mattress sheets every eight years due to the fact it will become too soft and disheveled which ruins your physique posture.

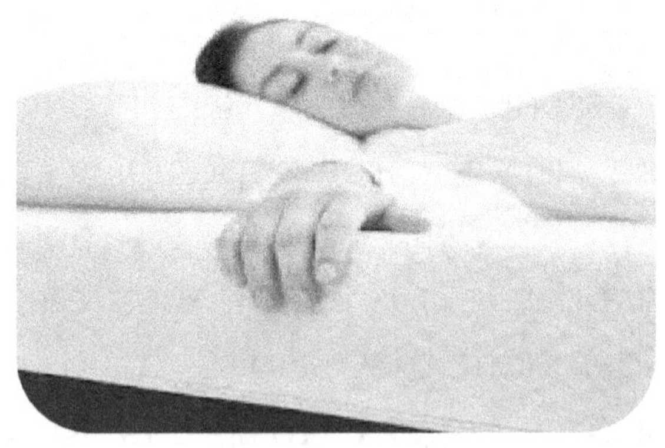

Tips To Purchase A Proper Mattress:

Neither too soft nor too hard, your mattress ought to be semi-firm. A mattress made of reminiscence foam is exceptional and cozy if you don't have trouble sleeping. And a little firm mattress will be exceptional if you hold tossing and turning while sleeping.

Along with proper vitamin and exercise, sleep is now regarded as an important contributor to good health. Lack of sleep and poor quality sleep make contributions to depression, terrible concentration, excessive blood pressure, and coronary heart disease. It is additionally related to mental illness, road deaths, and decreased productiveness costing an estimated $5 billion yearly (Sleep Health Foundation) to the Australian economy.

Research suggests that around 1 in three Australians go through from bad exceptional sleep and one essential aspect that contributes to a correct night's sleep is the proper mattress. Considering we spend around one-third of our life in mattress it is well worth doing some lookup into getting it right.

The proper mattress desires to be satisfied whist nevertheless being company ample to supply good postural alignment. Its length has to be at least 15cm longer than the tallest person using the bed. This capacity that you need to attempt the mattress in save and both you and your partner must be content material that the mattress provides comfort and support. This may additionally be complicated for some couples who differ significantly in weight. Some mattress fashions come with differing relief layers on every side of the mattress and this may additionally be a manageable choice for such couples.

7.   A Phone Case

A smartphone case is a must. Don't strive to save your cash on this accessory. People can easily see and observe how it looks, a dirty and outdated cover can decrease your standard. So, don't even assume of saving cash on this product. Also, presently a huge vary of mobile covers are accessible in the market, you can go and select the quality for you.

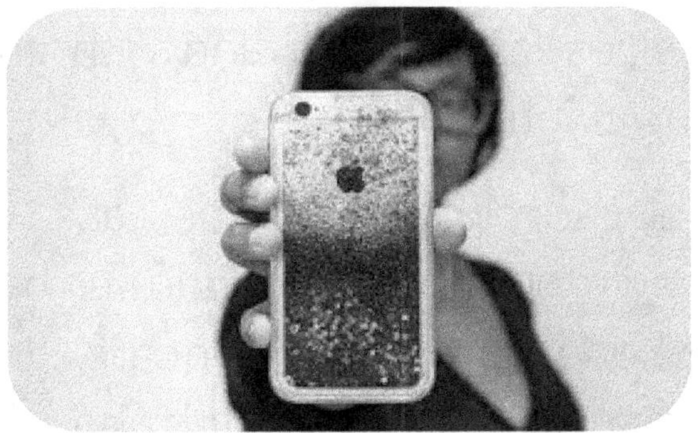

One of the most obvious reasons as to why a telephone case is essential is to shield your device's exterior. Smartphones currently are now not lower-priced and it is even greater highly-priced to ship the telephone in to repair. A cellphone case can assist save you time and money, whilst preserving your smartphone looking clean out of the box

Nothing can damper a proper day out like breaking your cell device. That's why it is so essential to use a cellphone case that protects from drops. But, it is additionally critical to use a grip accent that permits you to take selfies less difficult and with greater manage over your phone.

For typical gadget protection, a case, which covers the corners, edges, and lower back of a smartphone, is your high-quality bet. A precise case will shield your telephone from scratches and take in influence in these areas when your system is dropped.

The pleasant you can do is maintain an inventory of smartphone cases and use every case with the matching dress.

8.   TOILET PAPER

It's higher to use a suitable and comfy toilet paper than to use a low-quality uncomfortable one.

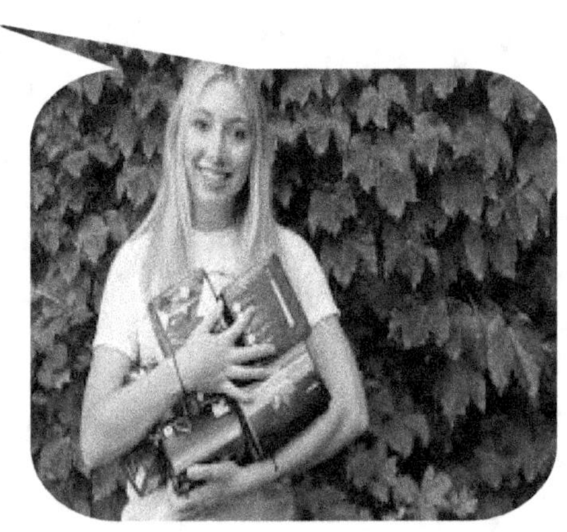

And wait, the price distinction between the two is additionally not much. Low-quality toilet paper is neither cozy nor useful. It includes detrimental components that can cause hypersensitive reaction or dermatitis. So take care of your fitness and from subsequent time purchase a little high-priced and healthful toilet paper.

Tissue paper products, which consist of paper towels and toilet paper, play an essential role in present-day life. They make a contribution to increased hygiene, alleviation, and comfort in our society. Tissue paper merchandise is notably engineered to grant strength, ultra-lightweight, softness, and absorbency, all at the equal time

9.   MAKEUP FOUNDATION

When it comes to makeup a self-aware woman simply can't comprise it. Makeup is vital and you must no longer spend less on this thing. Avoid the use of low-quality merchandise and begin the usage of nice merchandise due to the fact they give higher results. A cheap foundation is unhealthy and unsafe for your skin. It can clog pores and make your pores and skin too oily.

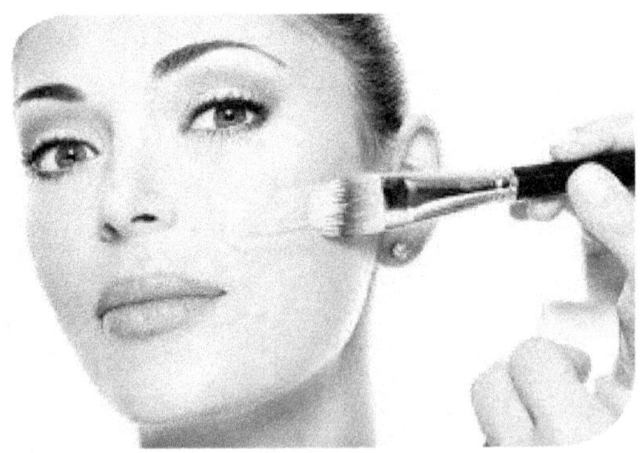

So why compromise with your face? Why take any risk? Go for high quality, appropriate makeup foundation for growing your complexion and to guard your pores and skin from damaging elements existing in low-quality foundations.

Research indicates there are two most important motives why female put on makeup:

Camouflage – Women who are anxious and insecure tend to use make-up to show up much less noticeable.

Seduction – Women who favor being relatively extra desirable tend to use makeup to be greater confident, sociable, and assertive

Makeup is supposed to enhance outer beauty without harming the skin. The pores and skin is the biggest organ of the body. It is a protecting shell that wants to breathe and be nourished and nurtured. As a section of each day routine, most females use make-up to decorate their appearance.

We discovered that, while makeup did make faces more beautiful on average, it only accounted for around two percent of the whole variation in attractiveness judgments. In other words, when someone makes a judgment of your attractiveness, makeup will only contribute around two percent of that judgment

Why girls love makeup? This is something guys maintain guessing about! Different varieties of women. Some hate the idea of simply a lip gloss, leave alone tonnes of paints on the face! And some in reality go gaga over the subject. Nonetheless, if no longer talking for all of you out there, I would like to factor out some simple fundamental motives as to why guys and not simply girls believe in the strength of makeup.

Why Women Love Makeup?

•   Many women discover makeup supplying a boost in confidence that helps the true feeling hormones kick in. At their location of study, work location, and parties, a little make-up now not simply heightens the glam quotient however additionally leads to a variable diploma of self-belief in women. This might simply be the application of a little mascara or even a lipstick, basis, and bronzer.

•   A lot of youngsters want to seem to be older. This is feasible with makeup that has the potential to seriously change that babyish face into a mature one!

•   Other the different side, ladies who have crossed the threshold of 30s desire to reduce their age. A range of cosmetics can decrease the look of wrinkles and fine lines to make them seem ravishingly young.

•   Women who find it tough to keep a healthful skin or aren't blessed with one can effortlessly disguise their imperfections. A properly concealer can cover blemishes, freckles, and darkish circles around the eyes. The illusionary impact can even down the problematic areas that make a lot of us experience insecure.

•	It's a great way to entice any individual with an instantly glammed up look. At times, what pleases the eyes, pleases the heart! Although that is no longer what all guys seem for in a woman, the degree or amount of makeup one prefers may additionally differ from person to person. Everyone loves a little attention. A sudden change in your look can flip eyeballs which feels wonderful.

•	It offers ourselves time, the 'ME' time! An all-natural look can be quite boring at times. It is enjoyable and a gorgeous way to experiment. If things mess up, you can begin all over and enjoy different looks.

•	To express what we sense like inside. A sexy look may make you appear outspoken or may also be blunt. On the other hand, a nude look might personify a subtle image.

The reasons for wearing makeup may also be varied. Nonetheless, that's simply the outer look and no longer what you are composed of on the inside. Keep the "YOU" real and that makeup will be an icing on the cake!

10. TAMPONS AND SANITARY NAPKINS

You can compromise with anything but with your hygiene? Never. Especially lady hygiene is a must.

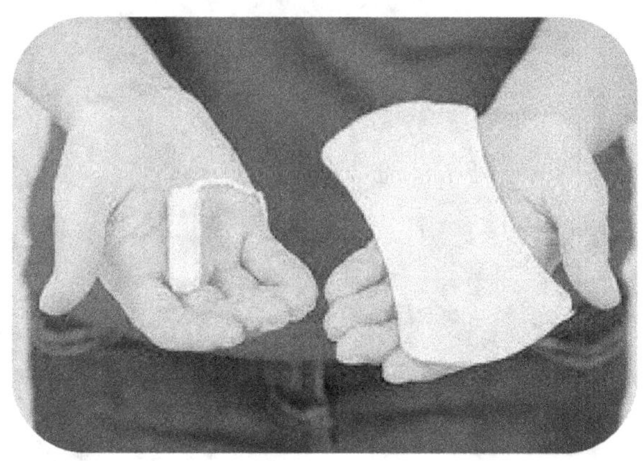

Always use tampons and sanitary napkins of top manufacturers due to the fact the usage of low-cost and low-quality sanitary napkins and tampons can lead to many ailments and additionally they are now not comfortable.

Before the disposable pad used to be invented, most ladies used rags, cotton, or sheep's wool in their underclothes to stem the glide of menstrual blood. Knitted pads, rabbit fur, even grass have been all used by women to cope with their periods

11. PROFESSIONAL PHOTOS

Taking selfies and speedy photos are okay however don't skimp on true quality image sessions. A professional photographer will make you appear even greater beautiful, stylish and he will seize you completely no longer simply face. So why now not go for picture classes regularly.

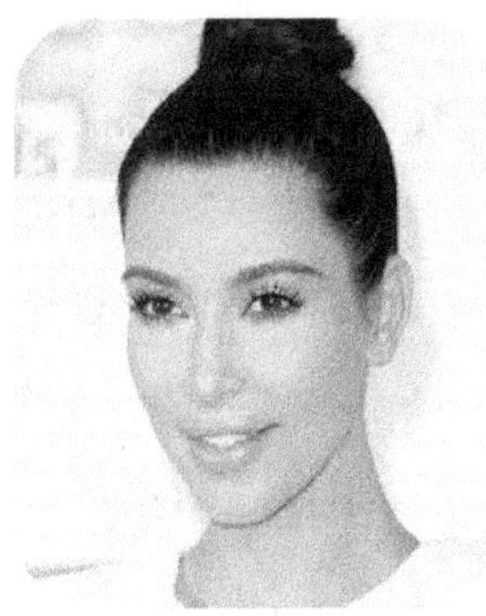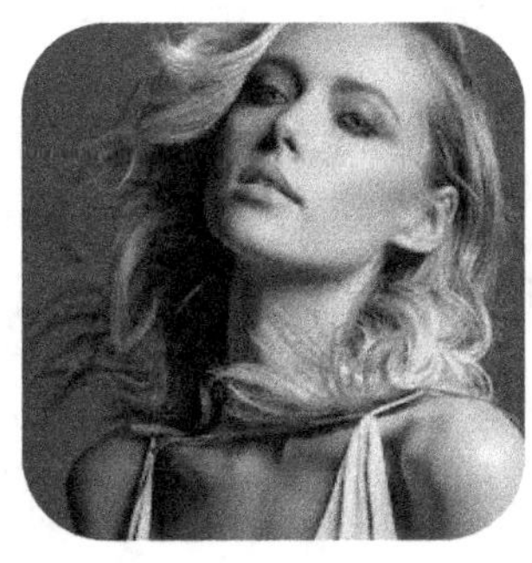

Photos tilt your recollections towards the good experiences you have had, truly due to the fact you are extra in all likelihood to take pictures of happy times. That's important, because due to a phenomenon regarded as "negativity bias," it is simpler to recall terrible times than good ones. Having snapshots of the latter keeps them vivid in our minds.

When you see something beautiful, it is natural to feel a desire to claim or even own it yourself in some way—and additionally to share it with others. Having images of things you love offers you the pride of doing that. On Pinterest, I love to acquire and share snapshots of fanciful tree homes and whimsical chandeliers. I get the pleasure that comes from searching at these matters besides having to own them (or purchase them, for that matter)—and the excitement of displaying them to friends with simply a few clicks.

12. YOUR VALUES

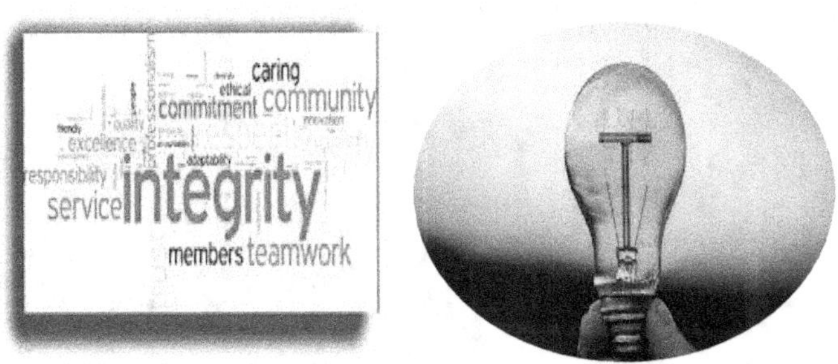

You must never settle for any scenario where the other person requires you to sacrifice your values to continue being with them. Negotiation has its place, however, the more you sacrifice on this front, to please them or hold the peace — you're enjoying with fire.

You shouldn't have to violate your morals to have a relationship. The right person won't even ask you to.

Goals matter, no matter what they are. Maybe you choose to lose some pounds, possibly you choose to get a promotion at work — something your intention is, don't compromise on it due to the fact anybody else thinks you should. At the end of the day, you need to be blissful with yourself, and you won't be if you derail your desires for any person else.

www.ingramcontent.com/pod-product-compliance
Lightning Source LLC
Chambersburg PA
CBHW070828260726
48654CB00024B/625